Implementation Fidelity of Infection Prevention Practices at Debre Tabor Comprehensive Specialized Hospital

Endalkachew Mesfin

Implementation Fidelity of Infection Prevention Practices at Debre Tabor Comprehensive Specialized Hospital

ELIVA PRESS

ISBN: 978-99949-8-977-5

Cover Design: Eliva Press
Cover Image: www.ingimage.com
Email: info@elivapress.com
Website: www.elivapress.com

This Eliva Press imprint is published by the registered company Eliva Press Global Ltd. part of Eliva Press S.R.L. Publishing Group

The registered company address is: Pope Hennessy Street Level 2, Hennessy Tower Port Louis, Mauritius
Eliva Press S.R.L. Publishing Group legal address is: Bd. Cuza-Voda 1/4 of. 21, Chisinau, Moldova, Europe

Title: Implementation fidelity of infection prevention practices at Debre Tabor Comprehensive Specialized Hospital, Northwest Ethiopia, 2023

First Name: Endalkachew Father Name: Mesfin Grand Father Name: Gebeyehu

Authors' affiliation

Department of Public Health, Wollo University, Dessie, Ethiopia

Authors' address

Endalkachew Mesfin (EM): endalkmes12@gmail.com

***correspondence author:**

Endalkachew Mesfin Gebeyehu

Email: endalkmes12@gmail.com

Po Box 83

Table of Contents

Content page

LIST OF FIGURES

LIST OF TABLES

Abstract

Background: Healthcare-Acquired Infections are a major problem in the world and within the healthcare delivery system. An estimated 5–10% and around 25% of hospitalized patients have healthcare-acquired infections in developed and developing countries, respectively. Infection prevention and control programs have proven to be successful in lowering the incidence and spread of infections. Thus, this evaluation aims to evaluate the implementation fidelity of infection prevention practices at Debre Tabor comprehensive specialized hospital in Northwest Ethiopia.

Methods: A facility-based cross-sectional design with a concurrent mixed method was used to evaluate the implementation fidelity of infection prevention practices. A total of 36 indicators were used to measure adherence, participant responsiveness, and facilitation strategy dimensions. A total of 423 clients were administered for an interview, an inventory checklist, a document review, 35 non-participatory observations, and 11 key informant interviews were conducted. A multivariable logistic regression analysis was used to identify factors significantly associated with the satisfaction of clients. The findings were presented using descriptions, tables, and graphs.

Result: The overall implementation fidelity of the infection prevention practices was 61.8%. The dimensions of adherence to infection prevention and control guidelines were 71.4%, participant responsiveness was 60.6%, and facilitation strategy was 48%. In multivariable analysis, ward admission and educational level had a p-value of below 0.05 and were significantly associated with the satisfaction of clients with infection prevention practices at the hospital. The major themes that emerged in qualitative data analysis were healthcare worker-related factors, management-related factors, and patient- and visitor-related factors.

Conclusion: The evaluation result of this study concluded that the overall implementation fidelity of infection prevention practice was judged to be medium and needed improvement. It included dimensions of adherence and participant responsiveness that were rated as medium, as well as a facilitation strategy that was rated as low. Enablers and barriers were thematized into factors related to healthcare providers, management, institutions, and patient and visitor relations.

Keywords: implementation fidelity, infection prevention practices, Debre Tabor comprehensive specialized hospital, Ethiopia.

Introduction

In healthcare environments, infections can spread from Health Care Providers (HCPs) to patients, from patients to HCPs, patients to patients, or HCP to HCP (1). Healthcare-Acquired Infections (HAI) are a major problem in the world within the healthcare delivery system (2).

The Centers for Disease Control and Prevention (CDC) define "healthcare-acquired infection" as infections acquired while receiving treatment for localized or systemic conditions as a result of adverse reactions to the presence of an infectious agent(s) or its toxin(s) within healthcare settings (3).

According to the National Infection Prevention and Control (IPC) reference manual of Ethiopia, the definition of HAI is an infection that occurs in a patient as a result of care at a healthcare facility or occurs if noticed after 48 hours of admission (4).

In 1970, the CDC introduced isolation precautions, incorporating policies and practices to prevent the spread of infection in hospitals. In 1985, universal precaution was introduced, and subsequently, in 1987, body substance isolation was introduced. Then, in 1996, standard precautions and transmission-based precautions were developed by the CDC (5). In 1996, the CDC coined the term "standard precautions" to describe a standard of care aimed at safeguarding healthcare workers and patients against viruses carried through blood or body fluids. In 2007, this was reaffirmed (6).

An Infection Prevention and Control (IPC) program was developed by responsible health authorities at different healthcare system levels to reduce the risk of HAIs (7). As a result, it was incorporated as a critical component of all healthcare systems, affecting patients, visitors, and healthcare providers (8). The IPC logic model was presented in Figure 1.

Infection management in hospitals began in the mid-nineteenth century. In the 1950s, however, outbreaks of staphylococcus aureus infection in North America and the United Kingdom promoted the development of contemporary infection control. This program has been part of the hospital's routine practices since it began 30 years ago (9).

Since around the year 2000, South Africa has had a well-developed national IPC program. Since 2007, the government has been steadily implementing national guidelines on IPC structure, standard and transmission-based measures, and outbreak control measures, with a significant reduction in HAIs (10).

Following the publication of the first national infection prevention guideline, Ethiopia has made significant progress in understanding and implementing evidence-based infection prevention measures in healthcare facilities. However, due to new scientific findings, the recommended evidence-based procedures are constantly changing around the world (11).

Healthcare-acquired infections have a major negative impact on the global healthcare delivery system, resulting in increased morbidity and mortality and excessive healthcare utilization (12). As a result, an estimated 5- 10% and around 25% of hospitalized patients have developed HAIs in developed and developing countries, respectively (13).

Despite infection prevention and control being the main agendas of the national or global health community, the third quarter report showed the implementation level of the IPC program at Debre Tabor Comprehensive Specialized Hospital (DTCSH) is low among the components of the Ethiopian hospital transformation guidelines and was identified as a problem by program stakeholders during the Evaluability Assessment (EA). Ultimately, it will enhance the implementation status by providing the intended information to relevant stakeholders who have already been identified during the EA. So these evaluation study findings will also be useful for policymakers, health facility managers, healthcare workers, and evaluators studying this program in the future. In this evaluation, the identified stakeholders followed the nominal group technique in defining the problem, formulating evaluation questions, setting indicators for evaluation, and assigning weights to indicators and judgment parameters for evaluation.

DESCRIPTION OF INFECTION PREVENTION PRACTICES

The IPC program is designed to prevent and reduce the spread of infectious diseases by any route to improve patient safety in healthcare facilities based on understanding the scope of the problem. To create a healthier and environmentally friendly healthcare environment, WHO and the states under its jurisdiction developed the IPC program. Healthcare providers and other concerned stakeholders must adhere consistently to the principles and practices recommended by the guidelines. For the IPC program to be effective, an appropriate structure needs to be established and strengthened at different levels. (11,28).

Program stakeholders

In October 2021, EA was conducted at Debre Tabor comprehensive specialized hospital. Based on EA findings, the main stakeholders involved in the implementation of the IPC program were Amhara Regional Health Bureau, South Gondar Zonal Health Department, Debre Tabor University, and Debre Tabor Comprehensive Specialized Hospital, Debre Tabor Town Health Offices, hospital workforce, and hospital clients and attendants. The identified stakeholders participated in defining the problem, formulating evaluation questions, setting indicators for evaluation, and assigning weights to indicators and judgment parameters for evaluation. An evaluation study findings will be provided to stakeholders through email, formal letters, and face-to-face communication channels. So these stakeholders were participated throughout the evaluation process, starting with the evaluability assessment.

Table 1: Stakeholders' analysis matrix for IPC program at Debre Tabor comprehensive specialized hospital, 2022

Stakeholder	Role in the program	Interest or perspective on evaluation	Role in the evaluation	Communication strategy	Level of importance(H, M, L)
Amhara Regional Health Bureau	budget, Supplies, Training, Supportive supervision, Planning and evaluation.	To know implementation status, best experiences and gaps in program implementation Use of finding for program improvement and decision making	Facilitate evaluation process Identify and weight indicators Set judgment parameters	A formal letter Email Through reading guidelines, policies	High
South Gondar Zonal Health Department	Supporter	Use of finding for program improvement and decision making	Facilitate evaluation process Formulating evaluation questions Select and weight indicators	Face to face presentation Email	High
Debre Tabor Comprehensive Specialized Hospital	Implementer	Use of finding for program improvement and decision making To identify strengths and weaknesses of the program implementation	Data source Formulating evaluation questions Identify weighting indicators Set judgment parameters	Formal letter Face to face presentation	High

Debre Tabor University	Supplies and training	Use of finding for program improvement and decision making	Facilitate evaluation process Formulating evaluation questions identify and assign a weight for indicators and set judgment parameters	Mail Face to face presentation	High
Debre Tabor Town Health Office	Supporter	To identify weakness and strength of the program implementation	Facilitate evaluation process	Face to face presentation	Medium
Hospital Health Care Workers	Service delivery	To identify a skill gap To identify the strength and weaknesses of the program implementation	Data Source Identify indicators Assign weight for indicators and set judgment parameters	Key informant interview Observation session/discussion	High
Clients and attendants	Service user	To get quality services	Source of information Formulating evaluation questions	Interviewer-administered interview	High

Goal and Objectives of IPC Program

Goal of IPC Program

- To improve compliance of infection prevention practices to 90% by the year 2025/26.

Objectives of IPC Program

- To ensure the availability and functionality of toilets, hand washing sinks and showers in all wards of the hospital by the year 2025/26.
- To decrease healthcare-acquired infections from 12.3% to zero level by the year 2025/26.
- To increase the HH compliance rate to 98% by the year 2025/26.
- To provide IPC training for all clinical and non-clinical staff, ad IPC education for clients and attendants based on the health education schedule by the year 2025/26.

Major strategies

- Ensure strong program management and leadership at the hospital level to oversee program implementation
- IPC education and training for all health care providers working in the hospital and clients
- Establish a robust HAI surveillance system at the hospital level
- Establish and implement strong monitoring and evaluation framework for IPC program
- Ensure and standardize the management of workload, staffing and bed occupancy in health facilities
- Improve the management and investment in infrastructure, equipment, and supplies in the IPC program

Program activities and resources

Commodities and supplies of IPC include personal protective equipment, consumables, cleaning materials and equipment: gloves, gowns, masks/respirators, aprons, protective eyewear (face shield, goggles), caps, protective shoes, detergents etc.

Supply

- Sufficient supply of all commodities and supplies for Personal Protective Equipment (PPE) should be regularly supplied for all staff.
- All fluid-resistant sleeve aprons, goggles and face shields procedure rooms

- Different sized and types of gloves
- Rubber footwear
- Disinfectant glutaraldehyde, Ethylene oxide, alcohol, a chlorine compound, H_2O_2, chlorhexidine and soaps
- Cleaning materials like different colours or sized buckets, laundry, mops and cloths
- Sterilizing materials, equipment, autoclave, oven, drum

The necessary infrastructure for proper hand hygiene

- Functional hand washing sink
- Functional water container(if there is no running water)
- Water tanker for reserve water during water supply interruptions
- Functional drainage system

Necessary supplies for proper hand hygiene

- Continuous supply of water
- Detergents(bar soap, liquid soap)
- Alcohol solution to prepare the alcohol-based rub
- Glycerin to prepare alcohol-based hand rub
- Personal hand towel/disposable paper towel

Supplies for Hospital cleanness and housekeeping

- Disinfectants and detergents, bleach, powder detergents e.g. omo
- Mops, cloths for dusting, brooms, soaps, buckets.
- PPE for cleaning staff and alcohol for hand rub preparation

Expected activities from healthcare providers

- ✓ Properly washing hands before applying necessary PPE
- ✓ Utilizing the necessary PPE
- ✓ Giving the right injection medication for the right person, the right dose and at the right time
- ✓ Properly utilizing sharp containers and other waste containers
- ✓ Disposing of medical wastes generated in the medication room according to the national medical waste management guidelines

- ✓ Ensuring proper documentation of activities in the service areas

Program results

Program outputs

- Number of functional toilets adequate for clients
- Number of functional showers available in all wards
- Number of rooms disposed of the medical waste following the guidelines
- Number of IPC-trained staff
- Number of IPC education given based on the schedule

Expected program outcome

- Increasing coverage of utilities
- Reduction of infection rate
- Improving the quality of care

Expected program impact

- Reducing mortality and morbidity rates by delivering quality care

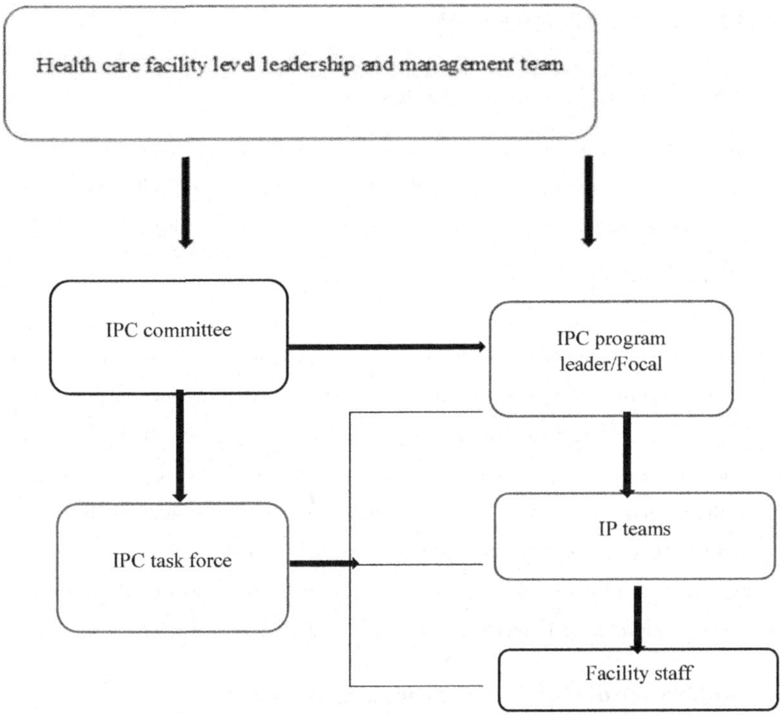

FIGURE 1: IPC PROGRAM STRUCTURE AT THE HEALTHCARE FACILITY LEVEL

LITERATURE REVIEW

Overall Implementation fidelity

According to a systemic analysis of hand hygiene fidelity implementation among healthcare workers, the most frequent unreported fidelity metrics were adherence and participant responsiveness, while the most frequently reported measure was quality of delivery (34).

An evaluation of infection prevention and control programs conducted in Indonesia in 2018, using qualitative methods, showed that the overall implementation of the IPC score was 39.8%, which is below the required standard (35). Poor adherence to standard precautions increases the risk of exposure to infections, so nurses should be updated regularly for better infection prevention and control program implementation in the facility. At the same time, creating a system to encourage role models to use standard precautions in their work serves to increase adherence, and thus improve the implementation status of the program organization must apply enforcement policies to maintain adherence to standard precautions (36). To reduce the risk of hospital-acquired infections, people's right to health, and increase awareness of health facilities' risk of infection, it is necessary to improve the implementation of IPC practices (37).

Adherence of staff to the national guidelines

Studies conducted in many countries revealed a lack of adherence to established guidelines for disinfection and sterilization. Due to a lack of compliance with guidelines and recommendations, enormous epidemics have emerged (38).

The evaluation of the healthcare workers' practices towards infection prevention measures in primary health care in Iraq revealed that the practice of HH was medium with a mean score of 2.23, the practice of PPE was medium with a mean score of 2.32, the practice of aseptic technique was high with a mean score of 2.53, and the practice of medical waste disposal was high with a mean score of 2.86 (39).

An assessment of infection prevention and control implementation at primary and secondary healthcare facilities in Nigeria revealed that 20.2% of facilities had an IPC program with clearly defined objectives and activity plans, and a copy of the IPC guidelines was available in 56.6% of facilities, but only 13.1% monitored the implementation of the program. 40.4% of facilities had healthcare workers who were trained based on updated IPC guidelines, 29.3% of facilities had sufficient PPE, and 46.4% of facilitated methods of healthcare waste disposal (40). An evaluation conducted in Singapore showed that the adherence to the use of protective devices was 83.4%, the disposal of sharp instruments was 54.6%, the disposal of sharp waste was 84.2%, the decontamination of spills and used equipment was 83.4%, and the prevention of cross-infection transmission was 73.5% (36).

In Ghana, an infection prevention and control assessment of fifty-six health facilities identified 34% of facilities with an IPC program with clearly defined objectives and 50% of facilities without clearly defined objectives, 50% of facilities had an IPC team, and 37.5% of facilities had senior leadership taking part in IPC related activities. In addition, an assessment of the environment, materials, and equipment for IPC in fifty-six facilities showed nearly 43% of facilities had water services at all times in sufficient quantity and accessible in all wards to staff, patients, and families. 50% of facilities, had alcohol-based hygiene solution stations but not available were at all times. And facilities having sufficient and functional toilets accounts for 41% of the facilities. While 82% of facilities have functional environmental ventilation in patient care areas (41).

A qualitative study done in Amhara regional teaching hospitals on IPC practice showed there was adequate information and IPC activities conducted in their hospital, but all participants admitted that non-adherence to standard precautions was prevalent and the majority of participants described facilities with a shortage of water or no functional water services at all, raising the issue of material shortage to apply infection prevention practices in some procedures, and HCPs did not follow appropriate standard precautions procedures (42).

Participant responsiveness

A study conducted in Egypt revealed that patients at Aga central hospital engaged in infection prevention practices with items like washing, using protective equipment and needle stick injuries; 98.2%, 96.9% and 68.7%, respectively (43).

Clients' culture and religion are critical to improving healthcare practice, so health facilities should respond to their expectations and needs by strengthening their understanding and involvement (37).

The patient's perceived satisfaction with cleanliness in a tertiary care hospital in Udupi district, Karnataka, showed the level of cleanliness of the surrounding (hospital premises, waiting room area, and corridor area) was 86%, 85.5%, and 90%, respectively. Level of cleanliness of wards: 86% of participants were satisfied with the ward area; 90.5% were satisfied with the ward ambience; 93.5% were satisfied with the availability of clean linens; 81.5% were satisfied with housekeeping; 93% were satisfied with utilities working, and 55.5% were dissatisfied due to poor cot conditions.

57% of participants were satisfied with the cleanliness of their bathroom or toilet area, 27% were dissatisfied due to bad odours in the bathroom, 99% were satisfied with the water in bathrooms, 31.5% with the means of hygiene, and 66% were satisfied with the floor conditions. 99% of participants were pleased with the cleanliness of the staff uniforms, and 97.5% were pleased with hand hygiene (44).

A qualitative study of barriers to IPC practice among Amhara regional teaching hospitals in Ethiopia revealed that HCPs are expected to give information or education to patients and their families or caregivers on how to prevent HAIs. But patients and their visitors have a poor perception of the hospital. Sometimes, health education might not be adequate to bring the appropriate IPC practice to patients and their visitors (42).

Facilitation strategy

Based on WHO's "Guidelines on Core Components of IPC Programmes', an assessment of the infection prevention and control system in Thailand showed IPC education and training for different groups of healthcare workers have been developed and delivered by health facilities and other organizations. There is also an incentive mechanism through a credit requirement for continuing professional development for licensing. On the other hand, standardized IPC monitoring and audits are often conducted by each hospital for its internality improvement, but no unit has responsibility for monitoring compliance with IPC guidelines (45).

On the other hand, an evaluation of infection prevention and control programs in sixty-five Austrian acute care hospitals using the WHO infection prevention and control assessment revealed that around 43% of the training for new employees, and at least annually mandatory training for all HCPs. 50 % of facilities established IPC training for administrative and managerial staff, 61.5% of the methods of IPC training for HCPs and other staff was only written and/or online form, and 38.5% was interactive training, e.g. bedside training and around 32% training was evaluated regularly, 35% of training was evaluated irregularly and the rest 32 % were not evaluated for effectiveness at all (46).

Conceptual framework: a conceptual framework for Implementation Fidelity (IF) of the IPC program. Having identified adherence as the focus for evaluating IF, for this study, Carol et al.'s conceptual framework for implementation fidelity was adapted because it is a comprehensive and useful way of assessing the IF of IP practices. The conceptual framework for implementation fidelity suggests that measurement for adherence (contents of the program) to the implementation is IF. It considers the elements' Strategies that facilitate the IPC program, socio-demographic factors and availability of water for hand washing as moderating factors of the fidelity level achieved. Adherence and moderating factors such as facilitation strategies and participant responsiveness were measured and given weights by stakeholders (47,48).

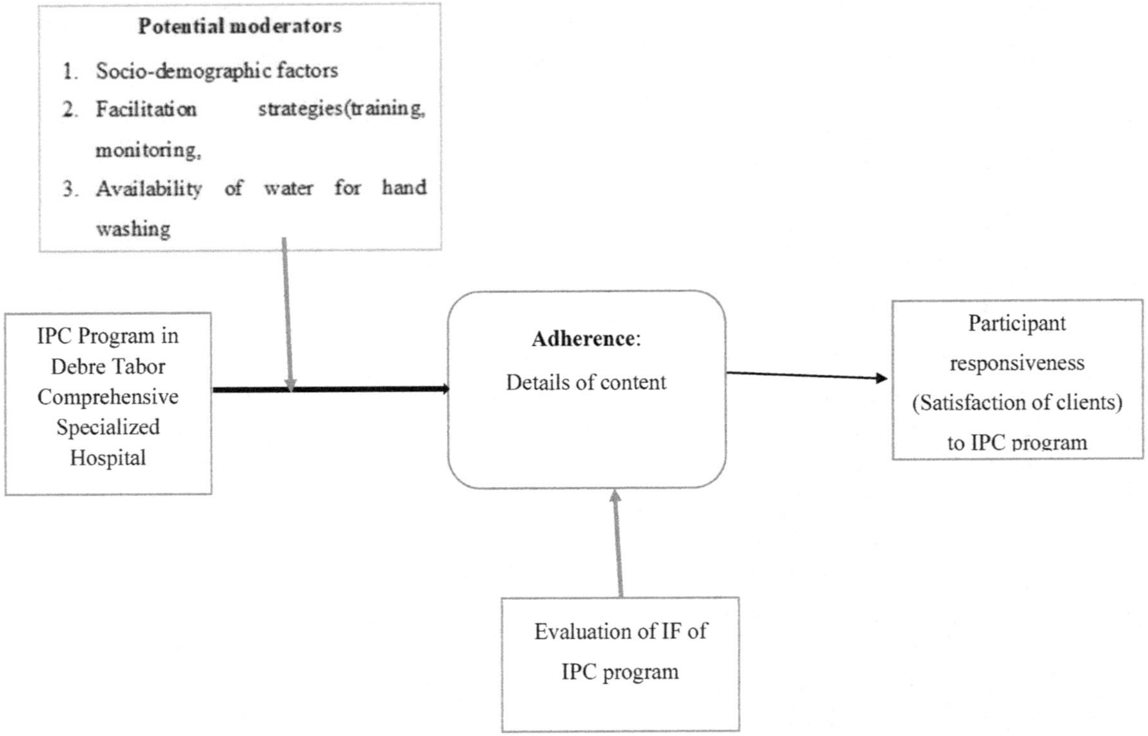

FIGURE 2: A CONCEPTUAL FRAMEWORK FOR IF TO IPC PROGRAM IMPLEMENTATION AT DEBRE TABOR COMPREHENSIVE SPECIALIZED HOSPITAL, 2022 (48).

Evaluation Questions and Objectives

Evaluation questions

- Do healthcare providers adhered with the guidelines in practicing infection prevention? If yes, how? If no, why?
- Is the IPP at the hospital responsive to clients' expectations? If yes, how? If no, why?
- Are the strategies of IPC in the hospital facilitating the implementation of the program? If yes, how? If no, why?
- What are the barriers and enablers of IPPs implementation at Debre Tabor comprehensive specialized hospital?

Objective of the evaluation

General objective

- To evaluate the implementation fidelity of infection prevention practices at Debre Tabor Comprehensive Specialized Hospital, Northwest Ethiopia, 2022.

4.1.1. Specific objectives

1. To evaluate health care providers' infection prevention adherence with the national IPC guidelines at Debre Tabor comprehensive specialized hospital.
2. To determine Debre Tabor comprehensive specialized hospital's responsiveness to infection prevention practices
3. To examine the facilitation strategies of infection prevention practices at Debre Tabor comprehensive specialized hospital
4. To explore the barriers and enablers for infection prevention practices at Debre Tabor comprehensive specialized hospital.

Methods and Materials

Evaluation settings and period

This evaluation was conducted at Debre Tabor comprehensive specialized hospital, which is found in South Gondar Zone, Amhara national regional state, Ethiopia. It was established in 1930- 31 by Dr. Ogambic, a Norwegian missionary. The hospital has been providing services for a population of 2,651,350.

It served as a general hospital till the end of 2019 and upgraded to a comprehensive specialized hospital in 2020. It is also 97km from Bahir Dar (the capital city of Amhara's national regional state) and 666km northwest of Addis Ababa (the capital city of Ethiopia).

The hospital is organized into wards for medical, surgical, pediatric, gynaecology, emergency, ophthalmology, and intensive care unit. It has a total of 125 inpatient beds in all wards. It has also hired a total of 534 people. Of these, 99 are administration staff; 16 specialists; 38 general medical practitioners; 05 emergency trained professionals; 11 health officers; 163 nurses; 38 midwives; 25 laboratory technicians and technologists; 31 pharmacists and pharmacy technicians; 08 x-ray professionals; 08 anaesthetists; 02 biomedical engineers; 08 HIT; 01 physiotherapist; 05 psychiatry; 05 optometry; 02 environmental health; 60 cleaners; and 17 other technical staff.

An Evaluability Assessment (EA) was conducted from October 15-30, 2021. Moreover, the evaluation was conducted from May 25 to July 5, 2022.

Evaluation approach

A formative evaluation approach was employed to evaluate the implementation fidelity of IPPs at Debre Tabor Comprehensive Specialized Hospital. A formative evaluation was used to understand what was done and what was not done, and to identify barriers and enablers to IPP for the implementation of the program. Since the IPC program was in the implementation stage, the formative evaluation was particularly important for this evaluation (17).

Evaluation design

A facility-based cross-sectional design with concurrent mixed methods was used to evaluate the implementation fidelity of the IPC program. A cross-sectional design was used to evaluate the implementation of IPPs at Debre Tabor Comprehensive Specialized Hospital. A cross-sectional design is composed of both qualitative and quantitative research methods that help to examine program implementation and answer the questions "why" and "how." The aim of combining the qualitative method was to strengthen the credibility of the evaluation findings and answer the evaluation questions. A concurrent mixed method was employed to triangulate data between qualitative and quantitative findings (18).

The focus of evaluation and dimensions

This evaluation focused on the process of the IPC Program, mainly the implementation fidelity of infection prevention practices and why and how the program was implemented in line with the national IPC guideline at DTCSH. To evaluate the implementation of the IPC program, the three constructs of adherence, participant responsiveness, and the facilitation strategy dimension of implementation fidelity were used. (16,19–21).

Populations and samplings

All clients who visit Debre Tabor specialized hospital; all healthcare providers and cleaners in Debre Tabor specialized hospital; the IPC focal person; all quality officers in the hospital; the matron; the hospital's medical director; and a hospital manager. The sample size for measuring the participant responsiveness dimension of the IPC program was calculated using a single population proportion formula. A 5% sampling error or precision at a 95% confidence interval and assuming that 50% of clients were satisfied with infection prevention practice are used in computing the sample size to achieve adequate precision (25).

The study's sample size was adjusted to account for the study population. The sample size was determined and calculated as follows:

$$n = \frac{(Z\alpha\ /\ _2)^2 * P(1-P)}{d^2} = \frac{(1.96)^2(0.5)(0.5)}{(0.05)^2} = \mathbf{384.16 \approx 384}$$

=384 + (384 *10% of non-respondents) =**423**

Clients admitted over 24 hours in all wards participated in the study. Sample sizes were calculated from the previous year's similar month's patient data flow (920), and the calculated sample size was 423. The kth interval ≈ 2. The first case was selected using a simple random sampling technique by lottery, and the subsequent cases were selected every two case intervals using systematic sampling techniques using liaison inpatient admission registration.

A total of 35 non-participatory observation sessions were observed. Eleven key informants (one KII with a hospital manager, one KII with a medical director, one KII with a hospital matron, one KII with the IPC focal person, one KII with a hospital quality unit team leader, five KII with ward coordinators, and one KII with cleaning staff coordinators) were interviewed. Resource inventories were conducted in all wards, rooms, and hospital procurement models using an adapted checklist. Twelve months' worth of documents such as the IPC Committee meeting agenda, IPC training registration, hospital quarterly review meeting agenda, hospital health education registration, and reports, were to exwase adherence and facilitation strategies from the period of July 1, 2021, to June 30, 2022. Assigned hospital managers, medical directors, matrons, ward coordinators, and cleaning staff coordinators who were working for six months and above were included in the study. Clients who were admitted to the hospital for more than 24 hours during the data collection period were also included in the study. However, clients who lost consciousness and clients whose age was less than 18 years were excluded from the study.

Data collection tools and procedures

A resource inventory assessment checklist was adopted to examine the infrastructure, resources, and equipment of the IPC program by referring to WHO infection prevention and control tools and national IPC guidelines (4, 22).

A data extraction checklist was used to extract data from documents (the IPC Committee agenda, the IPC training registration agenda, the hospital quarterly performance review agenda, the hospital health education registration, and the IPC supply procurement models) and was adopted by referring to the National IPC guidelines (27). A structured observation checklist was prepared to assess the adherence of healthcare providers' infection prevention practices to guidelines by referring to literature and the CDC Infection Prevention and Control Assessment Tool (23, 28). A structured interviewer-administered questionnaire to national guidelines includes the following: socio-demographic characteristics of clients, infection prevention practices of clients, and satisfaction (29, 30). A semi-structured key informant interview guide was prepared and contains the following: the backgrounds of the interviewee; information related to program management; strategies used to facilitate the IPC program; IPC training, activities, and training materials; IPC monitoring, feedback, and evaluation; and barriers and enablers to implementing the IPC program. A tool was prepared by referring to different guidelines and national IPC guidelines (22, 31).

Data quality assurance

For quantitative data, a pre-test was done among 21 clients in the Debre Tabor Health Center to check the quality of the data collection tools. And then a correction was made based on the pre-test findings. The data collection tool contained the clients' responsiveness dimension of implementation fidelity. Data collectors were supervised daily, and the questionnaires were checked for consistency and completeness of data after being sent from the data collectors to the principal evaluator.

Data management and analysis

Completed data were checked for completeness and consistency, and it was cleaned. Then the quantitative data was downloaded from Kobo Tool Box software and imported into SPSS version 25 for analysis. For qualitative data, field notes and audio recordings were taken and transcribed every night before being analyzed using open code software version 4.02 software. Data cleaning was done by the principal evaluator after it was sent from the data collectors. For quantitative data, descriptive statistics (univariate analysis) were used to determine the frequency, mean, and proportion of variables. A binary logistic model was fitted. Variables having a p-value of less than 0.25 were candidates for multivariate analysis. In multivariable analysis, a p-value of less than 0.05 with a 95% confidence interval was taken as a factor that acts as a barrier and an enabler of participants' responsiveness to the program. Participants' responsiveness (satisfaction) was measured using a Likert scale (1 = very poor, 2 = poor, 3 = good, 4 = very good, and 5 = excellent) of alternatives. Each satisfaction from the 5-point Likert scale of total items was categorized into two (below the cut-off point dissatisfied and above the cut-off satisfied) using the demarcation threshold formula [(total highest score- total lowest score)/2] + total lowest score. Each satisfaction item was analyzed for frequency, mean, and standard deviation.

Qualitative data were transcribed, coded, thematized, and categorized using open-source software.

Indicators/Variables

Indicators

A total of 36 indicators were used under 3 dimensions of evaluation 14 for adherence, 12 for participant responsiveness and 10 for facilitation strategy. These indicators were agreed upon by major stakeholders for measuring the implementation of the program and constructing criteria that judged the program's level of implementation during EA. The indicators were adapted from national IPC manuals, WHO IPC guidelines and literature (33,39,54).

Adherence indicators (14 indicators)

- ✓ Proportion of functional hand hygiene facilities in the hospital.
- ✓ Proportion of toilets with functional hand hygiene facilities in the hospital
- ✓ Proportion of HCPs adhered with respiratory source control measures
- ✓ Proportion of HCPs who offered facemask to coughing patients
- ✓ Proportion of HCPs washed their hands before contacting a patient
- ✓ Proportion of HCPs washed their hands after contact with the patient
- ✓ Proportion of HCPs who wore a mask during observation
- ✓ Proportion of HCPs prepared injections using aseptic technique
- ✓ Proportion of HCPs disposed of all sharps in a safety box immediately after injection
- ✓ proportion of HCPs adhered with single patient use devices for a single patient
- ✓ Proportion of HCPs record injections administered
- ✓ Proportion of HCPs adhered with work practice control measures
- ✓ Proportion of HCPs used three-bin to segregate wastes
- ✓ Proportion of cleaners engaged in environmental cleaning by wearing the necessary PPE

Participant responsiveness indicators (12 indicators)

- ✓ proportion of patients received education on how to prevent HAIs by healthcare providers
- ✓ proportion of patients who wore a face mask during the interview

- ✓ proportion of patients who washed their hands with soap and water in the hospital
- ✓ proportion of patients who avoid touching waste containers without wearing a glove
- ✓ proportion of patients apply sanitizer to reduce the risk of infection
- ✓ proportion of patients who discard wastes in the black colored waste container
- ✓ proportion of patients satisfied with the cleanness of toilets
- ✓ Proportion of patients satisfied with the cleanness of hospital compound
- ✓ Proportion of patients satisfied with the cleanness of hospital rooms
- ✓ Proportion of patients satisfied with cleanness of hospital beds
- ✓ Proportion of patients satisfied with food hygiene served by the hospital
- ✓ Proportion of patients satisfied with the cleanness of bed Lenin of the hospital

Facilitation strategies' indicators (10 indicators)

- ✓ Proportion of cleaners received IPC training in the first round of a year
- ✓ Proportion of cleaners received IPC training in the second round in a year
- ✓ Proportion of HCPs received IPC training in the first round in a year
- ✓ Proportion of HCPs received IPC Training in the second round in a year
- ✓ Proportion of monthly meetings conducted by IPC committee in a year
- ✓ Proportion of performance evaluation conducted by the hospital in a year
- ✓ Proportion of health education given about IPC in a year
- ✓ proportion of hand hygiene assessments conducted by the hospital in a year
- ✓ proportion of wards had IPC guidelines in their working areas
- ✓ proportion of wards posted hand hygiene posters in hand hygiene stations

Variables

Dependent variables: participants' responsiveness (satisfaction of clients) to the IPC program

Independent variables:

- Socio-demographic variables (age, sex, educational level. Marital status, wealth status)
- availability of Hand washing facilities

Operational definitions

Adherence was used to measure the compliance of healthcare providers to infection prevention and control guidelines through the inventory checklist and non-participatory observation. We used 14 indicators to assess this, with a 30% weighting.

The strategy the hospital followed to facilitate IPC implementation was IPC training, monitoring, and feedback delivered to cleaning staff and healthcare providers to enhance the implementation of the IPC. To measure this, we used 10 indicators and gave them a weight of 25% by reviewing 48 documents.

Participant responsiveness of clients was measured by both practices of infection prevention and satisfaction with the cleanliness of the hospital using 12 indicators and had a weighted value of 35%. Satisfaction assessed how clients react to the infection prevention practices and their satisfaction was measured using a five-point Likert scale (1 = very poor, 2 = poor, 3 = good, 4 = very good, and 5 = excellent).

Participant responsiveness (client satisfaction) was the outcome variable. Clients' overall satisfaction was dichotomized into satisfied and dissatisfied depending on the threshold, which was computed using the demarcation threshold formula: $\left[\frac{total\ highest\ score - total\ lowest\ score}{2}\right] + total\ lowest\ score$.

The independent variables of participant responsiveness were socio-demographic variables (age, sex, educational level, marital status, and family income) and the availability of hand-washing facilities.

The overall implementation fidelity of infection prevention practice was measured using 36 indicators over the three dimensions (adherence, participant responsiveness, and facilitation strategy) of fidelity. The status of infection prevention implementation was categorized and rated below 50 as low, 50–75 as medium, and ≥ 75 as high by program stakeholders.

Indicators were adapted from national and WHO IPC guidelines, and for each indicator, a score was calculated using the formula: $indicator\ score = \frac{Observed\ number \times}{indicator\ weight} 100$.

Judgment Matrix of Analysis

The judgment parameters were determined based on the calculated indicator score adapted from measuring the implementation fidelity of the student affairs program (32). The adherence, participant responsiveness, facilitation strategy dimensions, and overall program fidelity were classified as low (less than 50%), medium (50–74.9%), and high (greater than 74.9%). Based on the stakeholders' agreement, the weighted value given for adherence was 40%, participant responsiveness was 35%, and facilitation strategy was 25%.

Evaluation dissemination plan

The evaluation findings were reported and submitted to the University of Gondar, the College of Medicine and Health Sciences, and the Department of Health Systems and Policy. Then the approved evaluation findings were disseminated to the Amhara regional health bureau, Debre Tabor comprehensive specialized hospital, South Gondar Zonal Health Department, and other stakeholders through different means of communication like face-to-face, hard copy presentation, and publication.

RESULTS

In total, 423 clients who admitted to having waited more than 24 hours were interviewed, with a 100% response rate. Thirty-five non-participatory observations were also conducted in five wards. 11 key informants were interviewed, and resource inventory and document review (from July 1, 2021, up to June 30, 2022) were conducted.

Adherence to the IPC programme

According to the results of the inventory checklist, the hospital had an IP committee, an IPC team, and an IPC focal person with defined and approved roles and responsibilities, but the IP committee did not actively support an IPC team.

This was supported by the key informant interview result: there is an IPC committee established from different professions based on the terms of reference of the IPC guidelines, but the committee does not meet periodically.

"The IPC Committee meeting was interrupted due to some interference, but there are rules or terms of reference set on the IPC guidelines. The meeting should be conducted every month, and it is difficult to say that it has been in the IPC Committee before, but it will be strengthened in the future".

[32-year-old male Public Health Officer on the Quality Team]

The facility leadership did not support the IPC program by allocating an adequate budget. The hospital has IPC guidelines consistent with national guidelines that include both transmission-based precautions and standard precautions under them.

Due to a budget deficit, the three key informants interviewed stated that the hospital administration has not allocated an adequate budget for the IPC program.

"Already, we have established an IPC Committee in the hospital. The committee plans and acts in accordance with its plans; however, due to budget constraints and other factors, we are not adequately supporting the IPC program."

[38 years male environmental health professional]

The water service in the hospital is continuously available at least five days per week at all times, and a sufficient power supply is available for pumping, boiling water, and sterilization of medical devices and equipment.

The hospital rooms were built with natural ventilators, but they had no mechanical ventilators except in pharmacy store rooms. The hospital also has different isolated rooms for cohorting patients with similar pathogens. Cleaning materials, e.g., detergents, mops, and buckets, are readily available for the cleaning staff, and personal protective equipment is also sufficiently available for the cleaning staff at all times.

This is congruent with the key informant's findings that "if there is not an adequate supply of inputs and materials, we will be the first victims, and patients and professionals will be harmed next to us." So we avail cleaning materials and inputs sufficiently."

[30-year-old Cleaning staff coordinators]

TABLE 2: AVAILABILITY OF IPC SUPPLIES AND EQUIPMENT FROM AUGUST 2021 UP TO JUNE 2022 AT DTCSH, JUNE 2022.

Checked by observation				
No	Facilities/equipment		Functional	Not functional
1	Toilet with Hand hygiene station		10	1
2	Toilet with no hand hygiene station		3	1
	Hand hygiene station alone		2	0
3	Autoclave or sterilization		6	0
4	Laundry		2	0
Checked by document review from august1, 2021 to june 30, 2022.				
	IPC supplies		Availability in 12 months of a year	Months of stock out in a year
5	Disinfectant	Bleach	11 months	1month
		Glutaraldehyde	Totally absent	12 months
		H_2O_2	Totally absent	12 months
		Hand sanitizer	10 months	2 months

6	PPE	Mask	12 months	0
		Gown	Availed 1 times in a year	
		Boots(rubber wear)	Availed 2 times	
		Eye goggles	Availed 2 times	
		Cap	Availed 2 times	
		Apron	Availed 2 times	
		Surgical and Examination glove	9 months	3 months
7	Detergent	Omo	10 months	2 months
		Liquid and bar soap	12 months	0
8	Cleaning materials	Mops	outsourced	0
		PPE required for cleaning	outsourced	0
		Utility glove	outsourced	0
		Bucket	Available in all wards	
9	Waste bins	Non- infectious (black colored garbage)	Available in all wards	
		Infectious (yellow colored garbage)	Available in all wards	
		Highly infectious (red colored garbage)	Present in surgical, gyn-obs and orthopedic ward	
		Safety box	no at all in the hospital	

As shown in the above table personal protective equipment mask, gown, apron and rubber wear, detergents omo and soap, cleaning materials like buckets, mops and utility gloves, and waste containers black and yellow coloured waste bins were supplied with no stocked out in a hospital. Caps, surgical and examination gloves and red colored waste bins were availed in an interrupted manner however disinfectants glutaraldehyde and hydrogen peroxide and safety box were not availed totally in a year at all.

A total of 35 observations were done on the practice of respiratory hygiene, the practice of hand hygiene, PPE utilization, safe injection practice, sterilization and disinfection of medical devices and equipment, practice of medical waste disposal and environmental infection prevention and control in Medical, Surgical, Gynecology-Obstetrics, Orthopedics and Pediatrics wards (5 observations on each category).

TABLE 3: OBSERVATION OF INFECTION PREVENTION PRACTICE AT DTCSH, JUNE 2022. (N=5).

1. Observation on Practice of respiratory hygiene among healthcare providers at DTHSC, June 2022.			
S.No	**Yes for Items observed**	**Frequency**	**Percent**
1	Posted signs in a language appropriate to the population served, with instructions to patients and accompanying family members or friends	4	80
2	Source control measures like covering the mouth and nose when coughing	3	60
3	Hygiene of the hand after contact with respiratory secretions and spatial separation	0	0
4	Restrict susceptible HCWs from entering the room of patients	2	40
5	Face masks are offered to coughing patients and other symptomatic persons when entering the room	3	60
6	Wear a particulate respirator and conduct a seal check before entering the patients room	0	0
7	Persons with respiratory symptoms are encouraged to sit as far away from others as possible	3	60
8	Remove respirator or surgical mask after leaving the room and place in a plastic bag	3	60
	Total	**18**	**45**
2. Observation on Practice of hand hygiene among healthcare providers at DTCSH, June 2022.			
S.No	**Yes for Items observed (n=5)**	**Frequency**	**Percent**

9	Keeps the nail short, clean and without polish	5	100
10	routinely washing hands before contact with the patient	2	40
11	Routine washing hands after contact with the patient	4	80
12	Don't wear wrist watches and jewelry	3	60
13	Keep sleeves short and rolled up	5	100
14	The liquid soap is applied	5	100
15	The hand washing process includes rubbing hands together, palms, backs of the hand, fingers and wrist	5	100
16	Hands are rinsed with sufficient running water	5	100
17	Dry hands with an individual towel or electric hand drier	3	60
18	Avoid recontamination of hands at switching of the tap	1	20
19	Wash hands for no less than 40-60 seconds	4	80
20	Put alcohol rub to fill the palm and apply enough hand rub to cover all areas of the hands and rub hands until dry.	4	80
21	Check hand washing posters are posted at a visible location	3	60
	Total	**49**	**75.39**

3. Observation of PPE utilization among healthcare providers at DTCSH, June 2022.

S.No	Yes for Items observed for each item(n=5)	Frequency	Percent
22	Wear gown inside the hospital	5	100
23	Wear gloves before any intervention	5	100
24	Wear gloves for potential contact with blood or contaminated equipment	5	100
25	Wear surgical masks during procedures that likely to generate splash of blood	5	100
26	Remove gloves that are torn, cut and perform hand hygiene before putting on new gloves	4	80
27	Wear protective clothing that covers personal clothing and skin	4	80
28	Change protective clothing if visibly soiled and immediately	4	80
29	Wear a mask to cover the mouth and nose	4	80
	Total	**36**	**90**

4. Observation on safe injection practices among healthcare providers at DTCSH, June 2022.

S.No	Yes for each items observed (n=5)	Frequency	Percent
30	Injections are prepared using aseptic technique in a clean area	5	100

31	Needles and syringes are used for only one patient	5	100
32	The rubber septum on a medication vial is disinfected with alcohol before piercing	3	60
33	Check for the integrity of the vial/ampoule for the following expire date, breach, leaks and any particles	5	100
34	Make sure the right dose, formulation and route used for the right patient	5	100
35	Don't use boxes that are open, overflowing or punctured. Dispose safety boxes when 2/3 full.	5	100
36	During injection, disposable gloves are indicated only if excessive bleeding anticipated	4	80
37	Don't disassemble the needle and syringe after use	5	100
38	Don't decontaminate the needle and syringes prior to disposal	5	100
39	Discard a needle that has touched any non-sterile surface	5	100
40	Collect used syringes and needles at the point of use in an enclosed sharps container that is leak-proof	0	100
41	Dispose all sharps in a safety box immediately after injection	3	60
42	A patient should be kept in the room for at least 5 minutes after the injection has been given	5	100
43	Seal sharp containers for transport to secure area in preparation for disposal	5	100
44	Record the date and time of injection administered	3	60
Total		**63**	**84**

5. Observation on sterilization and disinfection patient care items and devices at DTCSH, June 2022.

S.No	Yes for items observed (n=5)	Frequency	Percent
45	Single use devices are discarded after one use	5	100
46	Reusable patient items and devices are cleaned and heat sterilised	0	0
47	Items are thoroughly cleaned and visually for residual contamination	5	100

48	Work practice controls that minimize contact with sharp instruments are used and appropriate PPE worn.	3	60
49	After cleaning and drying, instruments are appropriately wrapped for sterilization	5	100
50	Sterile and soiled devices should not be transported together	5	100
51	After sterilization, devices and instruments are stored so that sterility not compromised	5	100
52	Sterile packages are inspected for integrity and compromised packages are reprocessed before use	5	100
53	Reusable medical devices must be thoroughly cleaned before sterilization	5	100
54	The instrument processing area has a work flow pattern designed to ensure that devices and instruments flow from high contamination area to clean area	5	100
Total		**43**	**86**

6. Observation on practice of medical waste disposal at DTCSH, June 2022.

S.No	Yes for items observed (n=5)	Frequency	Percent
55	Use a three bin system to segregate waste into separate bins	3	60
56	The healthcare workers who generates the waste should segregate it where it is generated	4	80
57	Use leak proof container with tight fitting covers for contaminated and hazardous wastes	3	60
58	Check if safety boxes are disposed safely during the incineration	4	80
59	The swabs and other contaminated materials are disposed of in red waste container	2	40
60	Non-infectious wastes are disposed of in black waste container	3	60
61	Proper disposal of liquid wastes check the presence of septic tank	3	60
62	Don't mix infectious and general waste during collection or transport	4	80
Total		**26**	**65**

7. Observation on practice of environmental infection prevention and control, June 2022.

S.No	Yes for items observed (n=5)	Frequency	Percent
63	Clinical contact surfaces are either barrier protected and disinfected with an EPA registered hospital disinfectant after each patient	4	80
64	For small spills of blood, body fluids and other potentially infectious fluids immediately remove visible material	3	60
65	For large spills, flood the area with a 0.5% chlorine solution leave for 10 minutes and mop up the solution	4	80
66	Medical waste handled and disposed according to local or federal regulations	3	60
67	Cleaning equipments that has been contaminated with blood or body fluids by soaking it for 10 minutes in 0.5% chlorine solution or other locally approved and available disinfectants.	5	100
68	Engaged in environmental cleaning by wearing appropriate PPE to prevent exposure to infectious agents	5	100
69	Cleaning should start with the least soiled area and extend to the most soiled area	4	80
70	Don't dry mop or sweep the class room	4	80
	Total	**32**	**80**

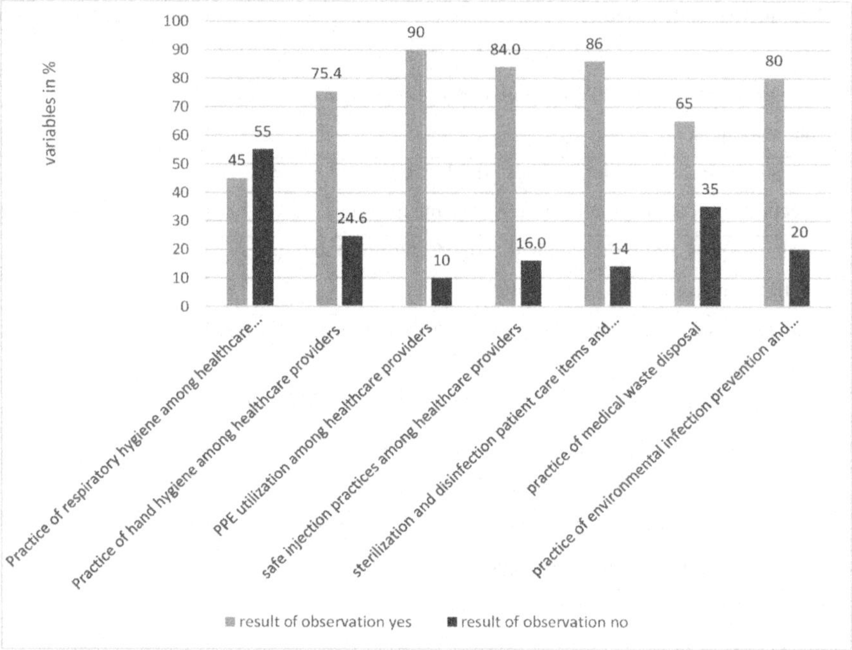

FIGURE 3: OBSERVATION ON PRACTICE OF INFECTION PREVENTION AT DTCSH, JUNE, 2022.

Healthcare providers adhered to the guidelines by implementing 45 percent of respiratory hygiene, 75.4 percent of hand hygiene practice, 90 percent of PPE utilization, 84 percent of safe injection practice, and 86 percent of sterilization and disinfection of patient care devices and equipment. On the other hand, cleaners adhered to the guideline in environmental infection prevention and control practice by 80 percent.

TABLE 4: SUMMARY OF ADHERENCE DIMENSION INDICATORS AT DTCSH, 2022

S.No	Indicators	E^a	O^a	W^a	S^a	A^a	JP^a
1	The proportion of functional hand hygiene facilities in the hospital	13	12	3	2.77	92	High
2	% of toilets with functional hand hygiene facilities in the hospital	15	13	3	2.6	86.7	High
3	% of HCPs adhered to respiratory source control measures	5	3	2.5	1.5	60	High
4	% of HCPs who offered masks to coughing patients	5	2	2.5	1	33	Low
5	% of HCPs wash their hands before contacting w patient	5	2	2.5	1	33	Low
6	% of HCPs washed their hands after contacting a patient	5	4	2.5	2	80	high
7	% of HCPs who wore a mask during the interview	5	4	2.5	2	80	High
8	% of HCPs prepare injections using an aseptic technique	5	5	3	3	100	High
9	% of HCPs disposed of all sharps in a safety box immediately after injection	5	3	3	1.8	60	Medium
10	% of HCPs adhered to a single-patient use	5	5	2.5	2.5	100	High
11	The proportion of HCPs injections administered	5	3	3	1.8	60	Medium
12	The Proportion of HCPs adhering to work practice control measures	5	2	3	1.2	40	Low
13	The proportion of HCPs used the three-bin system to segregate wastes	5	3	4	2.4	60	Medium
14	Proportion of cleaners engaged in environmental cleaning by wearing appropriate PPE	5	5	3	3	100	High
	Overall			40	28.6	71.4	Medium

E^a Expected, O^a Observed, W^a Weight, S^a Score, A^a Achievement in percentage(S/W*100), JP^a, Judgment Parameter

Participant responsiveness of IPC Program

Participant responsiveness of the IPC Program

Socio-demographic characteristics of respondents

Table 3 shows the socio-demographic characteristics of clients who participated in the responsiveness dimension of fidelity. More than half of the respondents (54.61%) were admitted to both pediatric and medical wards almost equally, whereas 2.6% of clients were admitted to the intensive care unit of the pediatric ward. Around thirty percent of study participants were unable to read and write, and 9.93 percent could read and write.

The age of the respondents ranged between 18 and 80, and the mean age was 34.44. Nearly 55% of them were female, and 51.06% lived in rural areas.

Of a total of 423 respondents, 80.14 percent were married, and the majority of them (98.35%) were orthodox. Regarding family monthly income, 40% and 4% of study participants earned in the range of 1000 and 2500 Ethiopian birr and less than 1000 Ethiopian birr per month, respectively.

TABLE 5: SOCIO-DEMOGRAPHIC CHARACTERISTICS OF CLIENTS AT DTCSH, 2022

Variable		Frequency (N=423)	Percentage
	Pediatric	116	27.42
Ward admitted	Medical	115	27.19
	Surgical	87	20.57
	Gynaecology-Obstetric	64	15.13
	Orthopaedic	30	7.09
	Intensive Care Unit (ICU)	11	2.6
	Unable to read and write	127	30.02
Educational level	Primary Education	119	28.13
	College and above	90	21.28
	Secondary Education	42	9.93
	Read and write	45	10.64

	≤34	238	56.26
Age	>34	185	43.74
Sex	Female	226	53.43
	Male	197	46.57
Residence	Rural	216	51.06
	Urban	207	48.94
	Married	339	80.14
Marital status	Single	67	15.84
	Separated/Divorced	12	2.84
	Widowed	5	1.18
	Orthodox	416	98.35
Religion	Muslim	6	1.42
	Protestant	1	0.24
	Farmer	208	49.17
	Government employee	69	16.31
Occupational	Housewife	47	11.11
Status	Merchant	32	7.57
	Daily labourer	15	3.55
	Other***	52	12.29
	Less than 1000 ETB	17	4.02
Family monthly	1000-2500 ETB	169	39.95
income in ETB	2501-5000 ETB	145	34.28
	Greater than 5000 ETB	92	21.75

Note: *** other includes self-employed, students, private workers and drivers.

Clients' infection prevention practice

Of the clients interviewed, around 22 percent got information on how to prevent HAIs from healthcare providers by using face-to-face health education methods (98.91 percent) and by using materials such as flip charts, brochures, and leaflets prepared in the Amharic language (1.09 percent). The majority (82.98 percent) did not also wear a mask or mouth and nose cover due to unavailability (43.30 percent), uselessness (29.63 percent), inconvenience (14.25 percent) and other (12.82 percent) reasons.

Around thirty percent of respondents did not wash their hands with soap and water due to the unavailability of soap. Whereas, nearly 5% and 16% of clients used hand sanitizer and put waste separately in prepared waste bins, respectively.

TABLE 6: CLIENTS' INFECTION PREVENTION PRACTICES AT DTCSH, 2022

Items	Frequency	Percent (%)
Do you get information on how to prevent HAIs from healthcare providers?		
Yes	92	21.75
No	331	78.25
If 'yes' to the above question which educational materials are used?		
Face-to-face health education	91	98.91
Using materials prepared in Amharic language (flip chart, brochure,)	1	1.09
Do you wear a mask/ a mouth and nose cover?		
Yes	72	17.02
No	351	82.98
If 'no' to the above question what are the reasons for not wearing the mask		
Unavailability	152	43.30
Uselessness	104	29.63
Inconvenience	50	14.25
Other*	45	12.82
Do you wash your hands with soap and water between activities?		
Yes	297	70.21
No	126	29.79
What are the reasons not for not applying the soap?		
Unavailability of soap	126	100
Do you prevent yourself from injury with sharp instruments?		
Yes	319	75.41
No	104	24.59

If 'yes' how do you protect yourself from injury		
By avoiding touching sharp instruments	296	69.98
By wearing gloves	23	5.44
If 'no' what are the reasons		
Lack of protective equipment	90	86.54
They have no risk	14	13.46
Do you use hand sanitizer to reduce your risk of infection?		
Yes	19	4.49
No	404	95.51
If 'no' what are the reasons not to use hand sanitizer		
Unavailability	317	78.47
Inconvenience	76	18.81
Other**	11	2.72
Do you put wastes separately in different waste bins?		
Yes	69	16.31
No	354	83.69
If 'no' what are the reasons to put waste separately		
Lack of awareness	343	81.09
Lack waste container	11	2.6

Note: other** = lack of awareness, negligence, religion and due to emergency, no importance, lack of awareness and due to emergency.

Among the total participants, nearly 5% and 77% of clients responded excellently and very good to the cleanliness of the hospital surroundings, respectively. Accordingly, less than 5% of clients felt discomfort, with a mean of 3.82 and an SD of 0.588.

Regarding the cleanliness of the toilet in the hospital, only 1.65% of respondents said it was excellent, but 15.37% of them said it was very poor, with a mean of 2.67 and SD of 1.135.

TABLE 7: LEVEL OF CLIENT SATISFACTION WITH THE CLEANLINESS OF THE HOSPITAL, JUNE 2022

Satisfaction item	Excelle	Very good	Good	Poor	Very	Mean	SD

	nt (%)	(%)	(%)	(%)	poor (%)		
How do you feel about the cleanliness of the hospital surrounding	21(4.96)	326(77.07)	57 (13.48)	18(4.26)	1(0.24)	3.82	±0.588
How satisfied are you with the hospital premises area?	20(4.73)	312(73.76)	73 (17.26)	17(4.02)	1(0.24)	3.79	±0.598
How satisfied are you with the cleanliness of waiting room area?	21(4.96)	259(61.23)	119 (28.13)	23(5.44)	1((0.24)	3.65	±0.671
How satisfied are you with the cleanliness of the corridors area?	19(4.49)	258(60.99)	127 (30.02)	18(4.26)	1(0.24)	3.65	±0.646
How satisfied are you with the cleanliness of the toilets?	10(2.36)	105(24.82)	128 (30.26)	95(22.46)	85(20.09)	2.67	±1.135
How satisfied are you with the cleanliness of hospitals?	11(2.6)	175(41.37)	207 (48.94)	26(6.15)	4(0.95)	3.39	±0.685
How satisfied are you with cleanliness of beds?	10(2.36)	198(46.81)	196 (46.34)	18(4.16)	1(0.24)	3.47	±0.630

How satisfied are you with cleanliness of linen?	9(2.13)	169(39.95)	174 (41.13)	66(15.6)	5(1.18)	3.26	±0.788
How satisfied are you with cleanliness of pyjamas?	7(1.65)	136(32.15)	208 (49.17)	66(15.6)	6(1.42)	3.17	±0.757
How satisfied are you with cleanliness of the staff gowns?	14(3.31)	199(47.04)	201 (47.52)	8(1.89)	1(0.24)	3.51	±0.607
How satisfied are you with hygiene of the staff?	15(3.55)	211(49.88)	188 (44.44)	8(1.89)	1(0.24)	3.55	±0.610
How satisfied are you with cleanliness of materials availed by the hospital?	12(2.84)	192(45.39)	206 (48.7)	13(3.07)	0	3.48	±0.607
How do you satisfied with the food services availed by the hospital?	4(0.95)	159(37.59)	239 (56.5)	19(4.49)	2(0.47)	3.34	±0.602
How satisfied are you with the information provided regarding waste segregation, norms of the ward	2(0.47)	69(16.31)	275 (65.01)	77(18.2)	0	2.99	±0.604

and infection prevention by the staff?							

Clients' overall satisfaction was dichotomized into satisfied and dissatisfied depending on the threshold, which was computed using the demarcation threshold formula: $\left[\frac{total\ \boldsymbol{highest}\ score - total\ lowest\ score}{2}\right] + \boldsymbol{total\ lowest\ score}$ (33). Clients' overall satisfaction was presented in table 6.

TABLE 8: SHOWS THE CLIENTS' SATISFACTION CATEGORY FOR EACH SATISFACTION ITEM ON THE IPC PRACTICED AT DEBRE TABOR COMPREHENSIVE SPECIALIZED HOSPITAL IN 2022.

S.No	**Satisfaction item**	**Satisfaction category(N=423)**	
		Satisfied (%)	Dissatisfied (%)
1	How satisfied are you with the cleanliness of hospital surroundings?	404(95.51)	19(4.49)
2	How satisfied are you with the cleanliness of hospital premises?	405(95.74)	18(4.26)
3	How satisfied are you with the cleanliness of the waiting room area?	399(94.33)	24(5.67)
4	How satisfied are you with the cleanliness of the corridors?	404(95.51)	19(4.49)
5	How satisfied are you with the cleanliness of toilets?	243(57.45)	180(42.55)
6	How satisfied are you with the cleanliness of bathrooms?	393(92.91)	30(7.09)
7	How satisfied are you with the cleanliness of the beds?	404(95.51)	19(4.49)
8	How satisfied are you with the cleanliness of the linen?	352(83.22)	71(16.78)
9	How satisfied are you with the cleanliness of your pyjamas?	351(82.98)	72(17.02)
10	How pleased are you with the cleanliness of the staff	414(97.87)	9(2.13)

	gown?		
11	How satisfied are you with hygiene of the staff?	414(97.87)	9(2.13)
12	How satisfied are you with the cleanliness of materials available at the hospital?	410(96.93)	13(3.07)
13	How satisfied are you with the cleanliness of the diet provided by the hospital?	402(95.04)	21(4.96)
14	How satisfied are you with the information provided regarding waste segregation, the norms of the ward, and infection prevention provided by the staff?	346(81.80)	77(18.20)

Overall, 348 (82.3%) clients were satisfied with the infection prevention practices in the hospital (Figure 4).

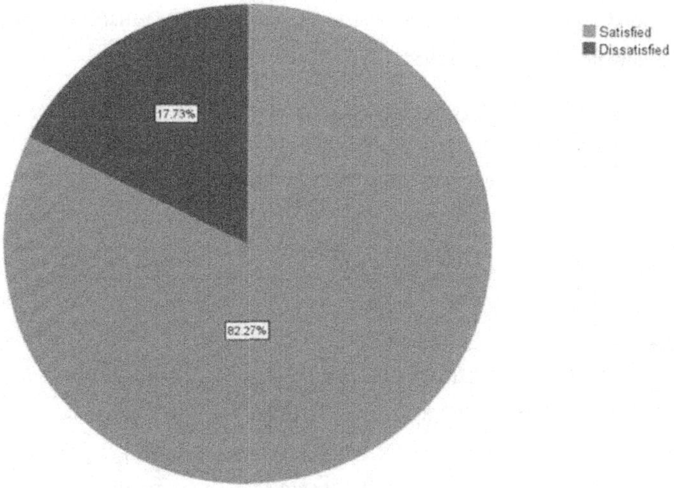

FIGURE 4: CLIENTS' OVERALL SATISFACTION WITH INFECTION PREVENTION PRACTICE AT DTCSH IN 2022.

Factors associated with clients' satisfaction with IPC practice

In binary logistic regression analysis, ward, educational status, residence, occupation, health education, and availability of water at the hospital have a p-value of less than 0.25 and are considered candidate variables for multivariable analysis.

In a multivariable analysis, ward admission and educational level (both with a p-value of 0.05) were statistically related to client satisfaction with infection prevention practices in the hospital. The odds of IPPs satisfaction among clients admitted to a medical ward were 0.36 compared with clients admitted to a surgical ward (AOR = 0.358, 95%CI: 0.165-0.777). The odds of IPPs satisfaction among clients admitted to the Gynecology-Obstetrics ward were also 0.32 compared with the IPPs satisfaction of clients admitted to a surgical ward (AOR = 0.315, 95% CI: 0.120-0.827). Moreover, the odds of IPPs satisfaction among clients admitted to the orthopedics ward were 0.12 compared with the odds of IPPs satisfaction among those admitted in a surgical ward (AOR= 0.117, 95%CI: 0.014- 0.940).

In terms of educational level, the odds of satisfaction with infection prevention practices were 3.5 when compared to the odds of satisfaction with IPPs among those who could not read or write (AOR=3.522, 95%CI: 1.574- 12.991). And the odds of IPPs satisfaction among clients who attended college and above were 3.1 compared to the odds of IPPs satisfaction among clients unable to read and write (AOR= 3.071, 95%CI: 1.638-10.119).

TABLE 9: MULTIVARIABLE ANALYSIS RESULT OF CLIENTS' SATISFACTION WITH IPC PRACTICE AT DTCSH, 2022 (N = 423).

Variables	Satisfaction category		95% confidence interval		P-Value
	Satisfied (%)	Dissatisfied (%)	COR	AOR	
Ward admitted					
Surgical	65(15.4)	22(5.7)	1	1	
Medical	103(24.3)	12(2.8)	0.342(0.26-0.313)	0.358(0.165-0.777)	**0.009**
Intensive Care Unit(ICU)	6(1.4)	5(1.2)	2.167(0.40-4.778)	2.302(0.035-4.621)	0.277
Gyn-Obs	56(13.2)	8(1.9)	0.411(0.196-1.169)	0.315(0.120-0.827)	**0.019**
Pediatric	96(22.7)	20(4.7)	0.618(0.349-1.397)	0.549(0.262-1.1510	0.112

Orthopaedic	23(5.4)	7(1.7)	0.116(0.015-0.902)	0.117(0.014-0.940)	**0.044**
Educational level					
Unable to read and write	112(26.5)	15(3.5)	1	1	
Able to read and write	37(8.7)	8(1.9)	1.59(0.152-3.648)	0.821(0.162-4.157)	0.812
Primary education level	104(24.6)	15(3.5)	1.015(0.589-3.907)	1.592(0.601-4.217)	0.349
Secondary education	30(7)	12(2.8)	3.011(1.559-11.589)	3.522(1.574-12.991)	**0.005**
College and above	65(15.4)	25(5.9)	2.912(2.032-11.399)	3.071(1.638-10.119)	**0.003**
Occupation					
Government employee	52(12.3)	17(4)	1	1	
Farmer	189(44.7)	20(4.7)	0.332(0.150-0.709)	1.098(0.321, 3.760)	0.881
Merchant	27(6.4)	7(1.7)	0.778(0.222-2.067)	0.838(0.234, 2.999)	0.786
House wife	37(8.8)	8(1.9)	0.672(0.164-1.474)	0.754(0.214, 2.659)	0.661
Daily laborer	7(1.7)	7(1.7)	3.13(0.789, 301)	1.901(0.231, 3.21)	0.999
Other	36(8.5)	16(3.8)	1.310(0.555-3.092)	2.519(0.847, 7.493)	0.097
Health education for clients					
Yes	75(17.7)	17(4)	1	1	
No	273(64.6)	58(13.7)	0.943(0.854-4.500)	2.156(0.879-5.288)	0.093

Water availability					
Yes	331(78.3)	56(13.2)	1	1	
No	17(4)	19(4.5)	6.593(0.547-8.720)	2.462(1.048-6.373)	0.052

Note other**=: 1=reference, COR= Crude odds ratio and AOR= Adjusted odds ratio.

Accordingly, the overall measurement of the participant responsiveness dimension was 60.6%, which was judged as a medium using 12 indicators (table 8).

TABLE 10: SUMMARY OF PARTICIPANT RESPONSIVENESS INDICATORS IN DTCSH, 2022

S. No	Indicators	E[a]	O[a]	W[a]	S[a]	A[a]	JP[a]
1	% of patients received education on how to prevent HAIs from healthcare providers.	423	92	4	0.9	22.5	Low
2	% of patients who wore a mask during the interview	423	72	2.5	0.4	16	Low
3	% of patients who wash their hands with soap and water in the hospital	423	297	3.5	2.5	71.4	Medium
4	% of patients who avoid touching anything without wearing a glove	423	123	2	0.6	30	Low
5	% of patients who apply sanitizer to reduce the risk of infection	423	19	1.5	0.1	6.7	Low
6	% of patients who discard waste in a black coloured waste container	423	63	2.5	0.4	16	Low
7	% of patients satisfied with the cleanness of the toilet	423	243	4	2.3	57.5	Medium
8	% of patients satisfied with the cleanness of the hospital compound	423	404	3	2.9	96.7	High
9	% of patients satisfied with the cleanness of the hospital rooms	423	399	3	2.8	93.3	High
10	% of patients satisfied with the cleanness of the hospital beds	423	404	3	2.9	96.7	High

11	% of patients satisfied with food hygiene served in the hospital	423	402	3	2.9	96.7	High
12	% of patients satisfied with hospital bed linen of the hospital	423	352	3	2.5	83.3	High
	Overall participant responsiveness			35	21.2	60.6	Medium

E[a] Expected, O[a] Observed, W[a] Weight, S[a] Score, A[a] Achievement in percentage(S/W*100), JP[a] Judgment parameter

5.1. Strategies and Factors of the IPC Program

5.1.1. Registration and report review

In the study, a total of 100 cleaners were employed in the hospital, but 60 cleaners were found at work at the time of the study because the number of cleaners had reduced from 100 to 60. All 100 cleaning staff received the first round of IPC training in a year, and 100% of staff followed the second round of training in a year. According to a key informant interview, all the cleaning staff received IPC training every six months.

"When we joined the hospital for the first time, IPC training was given to us initially. Then, every six months, we all go through IPC training. [30-year-old male, grade 10-cleaning staff]

Of 375 healthcare providers, 80 (21.33%) and 10 (2.67%) were trained on IPC for the first time and for the second time in a year, from August 1, 2021, to June 30, 2022, in the hospital, respectively. The majority of the healthcare workers have not received the training, as indicated by most key informants. "M*ost of us did not get IPC training, including me. It is better to say no trained healthcare providers". [A 29-year-old male BSc Nurse Professional]*

According to the IPC committee meeting agenda review, there was a schedule to conduct IPC meetings every month by the IPC committee. From the twelve times the committee expected to meet in a year, they met four times (33.33%). The agenda for the hospital's quarterly review meeting was reviewed, and the hospital's performance should be evaluated every quarter rather than four times (75% of the time) in a year.

As reported by all interviewees, the IPC program was monitored and evaluated separately by the IPC Committee and with other activities every month and every quarter, respectively.

"First, an IPC performance plan will be prepared, and then the activities will be monitored and evaluated in accordance with the plan by the IPC Committee during its monthly meeting. And it will be evaluated also jointly with other activities, but we are not meeting based on the schedule".

[35 years male general physician]

48 sessions of health education should be delivered to clients about IPC from August 1, 2021, to June 30, 2022. It was given four times to 240 males and 180 females, for a total of 420 clients and visitors, based on the review of the health education package in the hospital and hospital annual report. In the past year, no hand hygiene assessment was done on healthcare providers.

Of the five wards, four had IPC guidelines in their working departments, and three wards posted hand hygiene promotion posters in their hand hygiene stations (table 9).

TABLE 11: DOCUMENT REVIEW ON FACILITATION STRATEGIES OF THE IPC PROGRAM IN DTCSH, JUNE 2022

Activities reviewed/checked on documents	**Required in a year**	**Achieved in a year**
The number of cleaning staff trained on IPC this year	100	100
The number of cleaning staff trained on IPC two times in this year	100	60
The number of HCPs trained on IPC this year	375	80
The number of HCPs trained on IPC two times in this year	375	10
The number of monthly meetings conducted by IPC Committee	12	4
The number of performance evaluations conducted by the hospital this year	4	3
The number of health education sessions about IPC given to clients this year	48	4

The number of hand hygiene assessments conducted by the hospital in this year	4	0
The number of wards with IPC guidelines	5	4
The number of wards posted Hand hygiene poster in the hand hygiene station	5	3

Eleven key informants—the hospital manager, medical director, matron, quality team leader, IPC focal person, coordinators of the medical ward, surgical ward, gynecology-obstetric ward, orthopaedic ward, paediatric ward, and cleaning staff responded to the interview, and no participant disagreed to participate in the study. Among the participants, all of them were male, and only one respondent was in grade 10, and the other had a diploma or higher in educational status (table 11).

TABLE 12: BACKGROUND OF KEY INFORMANT INTERVIEWEES AT DTCSH, JUNE 2022

Profession	**Sex**	**Educational level**	**Number of participants**	**IPC training status**				**Ave. service years**
				Untrained	Only Onsite	Only Offsite	both	
Nurse	Male	Diploma=01 1st degree=05	06	04	02	0	0	2.42 years
Environmental Health	Male	2nd degree	02	0	0	0	02	2.25 years
Doctor	Male	1st degree	01	0	0	0	01	2 years
Health Officer	Male	2nd degree	01	0	01	0	0	4 years
Cleaner	Male	Grade 10	01	0	01	0	0	2 years
Total			11	04	04	0	03	

Barriers and enablers of infection prevention and control practices

The major themes that emerged in the qualitative data analysis were healthcare worker-related factors, institutionally-related factors, management-related factors, and patient- and visitor-related factors.

Healthcare workers' related factor

As described by some participants, professionals' awareness of infection prevention and control was poor, and they had poor utilization of provided resources. But there are no factors mentioned as enabling factors on the healthcare providers' side.

"The healthcare providers' awareness of IPC practice was poor." (26-year-old male, environmental health). "The problem with health care providers' attitude is huge." (32-year-old male, health officer). "There is a problem with professional IPC supply utilization as an owner" (38-year-old male, environmental health).

Institutional related factors

The unavailability of facilities such as insufficient showers and hand hygiene stations and some old buildings that are not comfortable to apply the current IPC hospital standards were the barriers mentioned as an obstacle to implementing infection prevention by almost half of the interview participants.

"There is one bathroom with one shower in the pediatric ward. There is a shower for the professionals. There is no soap for the attendees; there is hand hygiene station in the toilet".

[34-year-old male, BSc Neonatal professional]

On the other hand, the hospital's trend towards better achievement in the national hospital competition was responded to as a good opportunity to practice infection prevention standards.

"Our hospital is in competition with the national hospitals, and this is a good opportunity for the health care providers to use this experience as a trend".

[35-year-old male, general physician]

Management-related factors

Most key informants described poor traffic flow management, inadequate provision of IPC supply and equipment, and a budget deficit for the program as the barriers to implementing the required standards. However, the management and matron were receptive to feedback.

"From hospital management to ward coordinators, answers to questions are enthusiastic."

[38-year-old male, BSc nurse professional]

Patient- and visitor-related factors

As pointed out by some participants, the patient flow in the hospital was high and was a barrier to IPC practice.

"There is a very high caseload of patients. It is a little difficult to give health education about IPC to every patient that comes because there is an incompatibility between case flow and the hospital staff. Healthcare providers became tired of delivering education to all incoming patients".

[28 years old male Midwifery professional]

The barriers and facilitators of IPC were presented in Table 12.

TABLE 13: BARRIERS AND FACILITATORS OF INFECTION PREVENTION PRACTICE AT DTHSC, JUNE 2022

	Healthcare worker-related factors	**Institutional-related factors**	**Management-related factors**	**Patient-and visitor-related factors**
Barriers	Negative attitude towards IPC practice Poor utilization practice Lack of motivation The number of healthcare providers and cleaners was low	Insufficient shower and hand hygiene stations, an old building, Shortage of inputs	Budget problem, Poor traffic management	high patient flow,
Facilitators	The presence of competition	The hospital trends in	Management is receptive to	

		national hospital competition	feedback.	

The hospital's overall facilitation strategy achievement was 48%, which is low according to the decision parameter (table 12).

TABLE 14: PERFORMANCE OF FACILITATION STRATEGIES' INDICATORS IN DTCSH, JUNE 2022

S. No	Measuring indicators	Expected in #	Observed in #	Weight (W)	Score (S)	Ach. In percentage (S/W * 100)	Judgment parameter
1	% of cleaners trained on IPC training this year.	100	100	2	2	100	High
2	% of cleaners trained on IPC two times this year.	100	60	2	1.2	60	Medium
3	% of HCPs trained on IPC this year.	375	80	1.5	0.3	21	Low
4	% of HCPs trained on IPC two times this year	375	10	1.5	0.1	7	Low
5	% of monthly meetings done by IPC Committee in the year	12	4	3	1	33	Low
6	% of performance evaluations conducted by the hospital this year	4	3	3	2.25	75	Medium
7	% of health education delivered about IPC to clients this year	48	4	3	0.25	8.3	Low
8	% of hand hygiene Assessments conducted by the hospital in this	4	0	2	0	0	Low

	year						
9	% of wards had IPC guidelines in their working areas.	5	4	3.5	2.8	80	High
10	% of wards posted the IPC hand hygiene posters in washing stations.	5	3	3.5	2.1	60	Medium
	Overall			25	12	48	Low

The overall implementation fidelity of the IPC programme is 61.8 percent, which, based on the judgement parameters, is medium and needs improvement (table 13).

TABLE 15: SUMMARY OF OVERALL PERFORMANCE IMPLEMENTATION INDICATORS OF PROCESS OF THE IPC PROGRAM IN DTCSH, JUNE 2022

S.No	Dimensions	Relative weight (W)	Score(S)	Achv.in % (S/W*100)	Judgment parameter
1	Adherence	40	28.57	71.43	Medium
2	Participant responsiveness	35	21.2	60.6	Medium
3	Facilitation Strategies	25	12	48	Low
	Overall Process of IPC Implementation	100	61.77	61.77	50-74.9=needs improvement

Discussion

The implementation fidelity of the IPC program was judged using the three dimensions of adherence, participant responsiveness, and facilitation strategies. In this evaluation, the overall implementation of the IPC program was 61.77% using predetermined judgment parameters as set by stakeholders. As a result, it was rated as "medium, indicating that the program requires improvement. The level of adherence to national IPC guidelines by healthcare providers was

71.43%, which was deemed medium. Client responsiveness to IPC program implementation was 60.6%, and the hospital's strategy to facilitate IPC program facilitation was 48%, these were rated as medium and low on the judgement parameter, respectively.

The hospital's adherence to the recommended IPC guideline was 81.8%. The hospital had an IPC committee, an IPC team, and an IPC focal person with defined and approved roles and responsibilities, but the IPC committee did not actively support the IPC team, and the facility leadership did not support the IPC program by allocating an adequate budget. This is due to an insufficient budget allocation by the Amhara regional health bureau and the lack of attention given by the government.

Furthermore, the hospital had an IPC guideline, a continuous water supply (for hand washing, drinking, and taking baths), and a sufficient power supply (for pumping, boiling water, and sterilization of medical devices and equipment). These findings were congruent with the assessment of IPC implementation in primary and secondary healthcare facilities in Nigeria: 80.8% of healthcare facilities had running water and soap in sufficient quantity, and 94.9% of healthcare facilities had hand hygiene stations at strategic places (34). One possible explanation for this similarity is that the IPC program gained traction in both countries.

Healthcare providers adhered to IPC guidelines by applying 45% of respiratory hygiene, 75.4% of hand hygiene standards, 90% of the necessary PPE utilization, 86% of safe injection practice, and 65% of disinfection and sterilization of patient care devices and equipment in the hospital. In disposing of medical waste, more than half of the recommended activities and 80% of environmental infection prevention and control activities were completed in line with the guidelines. More than half of the recommended activities and 80% of environmental infection prevention and control activities were carried out in accordance with the guidelines when disposing of medical waste (4, 27). Compared to the study conducted in Iraq, the practice of hand hygiene, PPE utilization, and medical waste disposal were lower in this hospital, but the practice of safe injection was higher (the practice of hand hygiene was 74.33%, PPE utilization was 77.33%, the practice of aseptic technique was 84%, and the practice of medical waste disposal was 96.33%) (23). The reason for this variation might be differences in the economies of Iraq and Ethiopia.

Generally, clients' infection prevention practices were low. 78.3% of clients did not have information on how to prevent healthcare-acquired infection; around 83 percent of clients did not wear a mask or mouth and nose cover; nearly 96 percent of clients did not use hand sanitizer to reduce infection; 84 percent of clients did not know how to put wastes separately using coded waste bins; and about 30 percent of clients did not wash their hands with soap and water. The national IPC guideline, on the other hand, recommended four components to the client empowerment process: patient understanding of their own role; client acquisition of sufficient knowledge in their ability to involve their healthcare providers; clients' knowledge and skills; and the presence of a facilitating environment (27).

Concerning the satisfaction of clients, overall hospital cleanliness was high, accounting for around 82 percent. And areas with the highest satisfaction gained from clients were the cleanliness of staff gowns and the hygiene of staff, both of which scored around 98 percent, and the dietary hygiene provided by the hospital, which scored around 97 percent. Toilet cleanliness was the least satisfactory area, scoring around 57 percent out of all satisfaction questions. The finding of our study was similar to that of a study done on patients' perceived satisfaction with cleanliness in a tertiary care hospital in Udupi district, Karnataka state, India, which showed 99% of participants reported that the staff's hygiene was clean and 46 percent of participants reported that the toilet needed more cleaning (30). This similarity might be related to clients' perceptions of congruency, even if the healthcare setup and services are not the same. Based on these evaluation findings, ward admission and educational status were statistically significant factors in the client's satisfaction with the implementation of the IPC program in Debre Tabor Comprehensive Specialized Hospital.

Clients admitted to a surgical ward were less likely to be satisfied with infection prevention practices at the hospital than clients admitted to a medical, gynaecology-obstetric, or orthopaedic ward. This might be the IPC program well implemented in a medical, Gynecology-obstetric, and orthopaedic ward compared with a surgical ward.

The satisfaction with infection prevention practices among clients who attended secondary school and college or above was higher compared with those who could not read and write. The possible reason behind this might be that being educated increases the ability to compare the services delivered at different setups.

The evaluation findings indicated that IPC training was delivered twice a year to cleaning staff by the hospital. All cleaners (100%) participated in a training organized for the first round, but only 60% of them were trained in the second round. This is because the cleaning staff number was reduced from 100 to 60 following budget inadequacy in the hospital. The findings were consistent with the national IPC guidelines. On the contrary, from a total of 375 healthcare providers, around 21 percent of them received training in the first round, and around 3 percent received training in the second round. This was minimal according to the national guidelines. These low-trained healthcare providers implied that the hospital's fidelity to its support implementation strategy was not in accordance with IPC standards. Like the study done in Ghana, only 35.7% of facilities and healthcare workers received periodic training related to new or updated IPC (35).

In addition, the national IPC guideline recommends IPC committee meetings be conducted every month, but the hospital IPC committee conducts meetings four times a year. And the hospital was evaluated three times at the quarterly review meetings in a year. The first quarterly review meeting was not evaluated due to the war of internal national crises.

Infection prevention and control were prioritized as a topic of health education to teach to hospital clients and visitors per week. However, the report revealed that the topic is given to clients and visitors four times out of a scheduled 48 times a year. There was an IPC guideline in all wards except the gynaecology-obstetric ward. Similarly, hand hygiene posters were posted in three wards: medical, orthopaedic, and paediatric wards (4, 27).

At Debre Tabor Comprehensive Specialized Hospital in Ethiopia, qualitative data analysis showed that the barriers to IPC practice in the hospital were HCPs' poor attitude towards IP, inappropriate IPC supply utilization by HCPs, and a low number of HCPs and cleaning staff. These were thematized under healthcare worker-related factors, institutional-related factors like an insufficient number of showers and hand hygiene stations, old buildings, and a shortage of inputs for IPC practice, management-related factors like poor traffic management and an inadequate budget, and patient- and visitor-related factors like high patient flow. These findings lend support to the step-by-step implementation of the IPC program. Facilitators identified include the presence of competition among wards, the hospital's previous trend in national hospital competition awards, and the hospital management's receptivity to forward feedback.

These facilitators, unlike those studied in Jimma's specialized hospital, had an adequate budget and constructed a new hospital building with improved, albeit inconsistent, water access and adequate environmental cleaning (36). In a qualitative study at Amhara teaching hospitals in Ethiopia, the barriers and facilitators to IPC practice were also thematized as organizational, healthcare workers, patients, and visitors (36, 37).

Limitations of the evaluation

The findings of this study were limited to Debre Tabor Comprehensive Specialized Hospital. Therefore, it may not be generalized to other healthcare setups. It also has limitations when compared to other countries due to healthcare setups, health policies, and other factors that are quite different among countries.

The other limitation of this evaluation was the hawthorn effect during observation of healthcare providers' practices towards infection prevention. To minimize this bias, the observation was conducted by hospital staff.

Conclusions

The evaluation result of this study concluded that the overall implementation fidelity of IPP was judged to be medium based on the judgment parameter and that it needs improvement. The implementation fidelity focused on adherence, participant responsiveness, and facilitation strategy dimensions.

The measurement of adherence was also judged to be medium, and the hospital had an IPC committee, an IPC team, and an IPC focal person with defined roles and responsibilities, but the IPC committee did not support the IPC team actively, and the facility leadership did not support the IPC program by allocating an adequate budget.

Participants' responsiveness dimension was judged to be medium. It included client practices for infection prevention as well as client satisfaction with hospital cleanliness.

Clients' infection prevention practice in the hospital was low. Client satisfaction with hospital cleanliness was high, accounting for approximately 82 percent. Admission to medical, gynaecology-obstetric, and orthopaedic wards and the educational level of clients were factors attributed to the satisfaction with the IPC program.

The measurement of the facilitation strategy was judged to be low, and it included IPC training that was delivered twice a year to all cleaning staff by the hospital. On the contrary, 21 percent of HCPs received the training in the first round, and around 3 percent of them received it in the second round. Amhara Regional Health Bureau better allocates an adequate budget for the infection prevention and control program, and the IPC program shall be considered during planning, budgeting, monitoring, and evaluation of activities, and the IPC program shall be incorporated into other facility routine activities. Debre Tabor Comprehensive Hospital is better able to deliver health education about infection prevention and control to clients to enable them to be sufficiently confident on their ability to involve their healthcare providers.

META-EVALUATION

While evaluations are used to assess infection prevention practices, evaluation by itself needs to be of good quality and must be conducted legally and ethically to increase the credibility of evaluation results. Four standards: utility, property, feasibility and accuracy with 30 sub standards that had 68 specific criteria. The overall evaluation of standards measured 83.33 percent which was very good based on the standards criteria.

Utility: All stakeholders like Amhara regional health bureau, Debre Tabor University, South Gondar Zone Health Department, Debre Tabor Comprehensive Specialized Hospital, Debre Tabor Town Health Office, and hospital staff were the identified relevant stakeholders in this program and they were involved during EA and proposal development stage of the evaluation study. Their concerns was incorporated into the document then the evaluation findings will be presented to them at the end. This standard measurement result was 73.7 percent.

Property: The evaluation study was conducted legally and ethically about the welfare of those affected by its results so to ensure this ethical letter was approved by Ethical Review Committee of Medicine and Health Sciences College from the University of Gondar. The result of property standard was 75 percent.

Feasibility: The methods, sequences, timing and procedures used in this evaluation study was realistic and applicable as well as the cost incurred was feasible. The feasibility scored 75 percent.

Accuracy: The accuracy of data was kept by using valid and reliable data collection tools during the data collection phase and by checking the consistency and complementarity of both qualitative and quantitative data during the analysis phase(64–66). The accuracy standard measurement was 92 percent.

Table 16: Summary of meta-evaluation standards result using process evaluation checklist for implementation of IPC program at Debre Tabor comprehensive specialized hospital, 2022.

standards	Sub-standards	Total number of specific criteria	Number of specific criteria met	percentage
Utility (7 standards)	Stakeholders identification	3	3	
	Evaluator credibility	3	2	
	Information scope and selection	2	2	
	Values identification	3	3	
	Report clarity	3	3	
	Report timeliness and clarity	3	0	
	Evaluation impact	2	1	
Subtotal		**19**	**14**	**73.7**
Property (8 standards)	Service orientation	2	2	
	Formal agreements	2	1	
	Rights of human subjects	2	2	
	Human interactions	2	1	
	Complete and fair assessment	2	2	
	Disclosure of findings	2	1	
	Conflict of interest	2	1	
	Fiscal responsibility	2	2	
Subtotal		**16**	**12**	**75**
	Practical procedures	3	2	

Feasibility (3 standards)	Political viability	3	3	
	Cost-effectiveness	2	1	
Subtotal		**8**	**6**	**75**
Accuracy (12 standards)	Program documentation	1	1	
	Context analysis	1	1	
	Described purpose and procedures	2	2	
	Defensible information sources	2	2	
	Valid information	3	3	
	Reliable information	4	3	
	Systematic information	2	2	
	Analysis of quantitative information	2	2	
	Analysis of qualitative information	2	2	
	Justified information	2	2	
	Impartial reporting	2	2	
	Meta-evaluation	2	1	
Subtotal		**25**	**23**	**92**
Total judgment parameter		**68**	**55**	**80.9** (very good)

Abbreviations

AMR: Anti-Microbial Resistance; CASH: Clean and Safe Health facilities; CDC: Centers for Diseases Prevention and Control; DTCSH: Debre Tabor Comprehensive Specialized Hospital; EA: Evaluability Assessment; EFMOH: Ethiopian Federal Ministry of Health; IF: Implementation Fidelity; HAI: Health care Acquired Infection; HH: Hand Hygiene; IP: Infection Prevention; IPC: Infection Prevention and Control; IPPs: Infection Prevention practices; KII: Key Informant Interview; M&E: Monitoring and Evaluation; PPE: Personal Protective Equipment; SDG: Sustainable Development Goal; SPSS: Statistics Package for Social Sciences; SSI: Surgical Site Infection; WASH: Safe Water, Sanitation and Hygiene; WHO: World Health Organization.

Declarations

Ethics approval and consent to participate: Ethical clearance was obtained from the University of Gondar, the Institute of public health, Ethical Review Committee. Official permission was obtained from Debre Tabor comprehensive specialized hospital to cascade data collection. From each participant has written informed consent was obtained as per Helsinki declaration. In each case, the purpose and procedure of the study were explained to the study subjects, and each was asked for their willingness to have an observation of interaction or interview with no need of telling and recording their name and conducted for academic purposes only. They were also informed that they have the right to decline or not participate.

Consent of publication: Not applicable

Availability of data and materials: data will be available upon request from the corresponding author.

Competing interests: All authors declared that they have no competing interests.

Funding: This research did not receive any grant from any funding agency in the public, commercial or non-profit sectors.

Authors' contributions: EM, worked on the conception of the research idea, designed the study, was involved in proposal writing, training and supervising the data collectors, and analyzed and interpreted the results. AD, LY SM, and KA played their role in critically revising the proposal, participating in the design, analyzing and interpreting the results and writing the manuscript. All authors were involved in reading and approving the final manuscript.

Acknowledgments: Our special gratitude and appreciation go to the University of Gondar, Institute of Public Health, Health Systems and Policy Department. And our appreciation also go to Debre Tabor Comprehensive Specialized Hospital staff, hospital clients and stakeholders for their kind cooperation in all issues. We would also like to thank the data collectors and supervisors.

REFERENCES

1. Government of Kenya. National Infection Prevention and Control Policy for Health Care Services in Kenya. 2015; 53(2):1–135.

2. Ali S, Birhane M, Bekele S, Kibru G, Teshager L, Yilma Y, et al. Healthcare-associated infection and its risk factors among patients admitted to a tertiary hospital in Ethiopia: a longitudinal study. Antimicrobial Resist Infect Control. 2018; 7(2).

3. Beyera GK, Beyen TK. Epidemiology of exposure to HIV/AIDS risky conditions in healthcare settings: The case of health facilities in Gondar City, North West Ethiopia. BMC Public Health. 2014; 14(1):1–8.

4. Prevention NI, Providers S. (IPC) Reference Manual for Health Care Service Providers and Managers. Vol. 2. 2019.

5. Tietjen L, Mcintosh N. Infection Prevention Guidelines for Healthcare Facilities with Limited Resources. 2003.

6. Columbia U of B. Manual of Infection Prevention and Control. 2021. 1–65 p.

7. World Health Organization (WHO). Practical Guidelines for Infection Control in Health Care Facilities Practical Guidelines for Infection Control in Health Care Facilities. Vol. 41, SEARO Regional Publication. 2004. 110 p.

8. World Health Organization (WHO). Guidelines on core components of infection prevention and control programmes at the national and acute health care facility level. World Health Organization. 2016. 91 p.

9. Ling Moi Lin CTY and SWHA. Infection Control Asian Healthcare Work for the Third. 2011.

10. Sastry S, Masroor N, Bearman G, Hajjeh R, Holmes A, Memish Z, et al. The 17th International Congress on Infectious Diseases workshop on developing infection prevention and control resources for low- and middle-income countries. Int J Infect Dis. 2017; 57:138–43.

11. Manual R, Service FOR, In M, Facilities H, Ministry F, Health OF, et al. Infection Prevention and Patient Safety Reference For Healthcare Providers and Managers in Healthcare Facilities of Ethiopia. Second. Addis Ababa: Federal Ministry of Health; 2012.

12. (CINQ) C sur les infections nosocomial du Q. Infection Prevention and Control Measures in the Emergency Department. 2013.

13. Sunley K, Gallagher R, Reidy MP, Dunn H. Essential practice for infection prevention and control: RCN guidance for nursing staff, 2/2. Br J Health Assist. 2018; 12(1):28–33.

14. Mr. Patrick Lynch, National Director QA and V (QAV). Patient Safety Strategy.

15. Komiyama A, Kato S, Ninomiya I. The Importance of Implementation Fidelity. Kaos GL Derg. 2002; 2(75):147–73.

16. Carroll C, Patterson M, Wood S, Booth A, Rick J, Balain S. A conceptual framework for implementation fidelity. Implement Sci. 2007; 2(1):1–9.

17. Carou-jones V. Formative evaluation of the UNFPA innovation initiative UNFPA Evaluation Office. 2016;

18. S.Wholey KENHPHJ, editor. Handbook of Practical Program Evaluation. Fourth edi. Canada: Wiley; 2015.

19. Project L. E VALUATION B RIEF 2 1 Evaluation Second Project Workshop. 2009 ;(October):1–6.

20. Assogba Y. The Importance of Implementation Fidelity. Arsyad, Azhar. 2002 ;(25):2002.

21. Pérez D, Stuyft P Van Der, Zabala C, Castro M, Lefèvre P. A modified theoretical framework to assess implementation fidelity of adaptive public health interventions. Implement Sci. 2016; 1–11.

22. WHO. Infection Prevention and Control Assessment Framework. 2018. 1–15 p.

23. Naji AB. Evaluation of Healthcare workers' Practices Concerning Infection Control Measures at Primary Health Care Centers. 2017; 1(2):63–8.

24. Fidelity MI. E VALUATION B RIEF. 2009 ;(October).

25. ACAR T. Determination of Sample Size and Observation Units. Int J Assess Tools Educ. 2019; 6(5):37–43.

26. Population F, Health M, Health C, Programs STD, Turner AG, Tsui AO, et al. SAMPLING MANUAL for FACILITY SURVEYS. 2001.

27. Federal Ministry of Health Ethiopia. National Infection Prevention and Control Training Participant Manual. 2019; I (October).

28. Prevention C for DC and. Infection Prevention and Control Assessment Tool for Acute Care Hospitals. 2016.

29. Mousad H, Abou E, Emad M, Hussien E, El S, Abd H, et al. Assessment of Patients ' and Visitors ' Knowledge , Practice , and Attitude Related to Preventing Infection at Aga Centralized Hospital. 2020; 7(1):429–47.

30. Kumar S, Tomar S. Patient's perceived satisfaction on cleanliness in a tertiary care hospital. Int J Manag Res Bus Strateg. 2014; 3:3.

31. USAID. Infection control assessment tool (ICAT): A standardized approach for improving hospital infection control practices. Management. 2013 ;(May):1–26.

32. Finney SJ, Ph D. Research & practice in assessment. 2013; 15–28.

33. Personal F, To P, Of C. Threshold Concepts : FROM PERSONAL PRACTICE TO.

34. Ct B, Tc U. Assessment of Infection Prevention and Control Implementation in Primary and Secondary Health Care Facilities in Rivers State. 2021; 33(2):100–14.

35. Oppong TB, Amponsem-Boateng C, Oppong EE, Opolot G. Infection Prevention and Control Preparedness Level and Associated Determinants in 56 Acute Healthcare Facilities in Ghana. 2020; 4263–71.

36. Kenzie M, Safdar N, Abdissa A, Yilma D, Ibrahim S, Siraj D, et al. Infection prevention and control practices in Jimma, Ethiopia. 1996; 1–9.

37. Yallew WW, Kumie A, Yehuala FM. Barriers to infection prevention and control practice among Amhara region teaching hospitals in Ethiopia: Qualitative study. Int J Infect Control. 2019; 15(2):1–8.

38. World Health Organization. Module 6: monitoring and evaluating an implementation research project. 2014;

39. Umhlaba Development Services. Introduction to Monitoring and Evaluation Using the Logical Framework Approach. 2017; 59.

40. MSF Vienna Evaluation Unit. Evaluation Manual. 2008; 68.

Publisher: Eliva Press Global Ltd

Email: info@elivapress.com

Made in United States
North Haven, CT
04 November 2026

21772741R00046